I Choose Me

A Woman's Guide to Better Health God's Way

Latasha Brown

Copyright © 2016
by Latasha Brown

All rights reserved. No part of this publication may be reproduced, distributed, or transmitted in any form or by any means, including photocopying, recording, or other electronic or mechanical methods, without the prior written permission of the publisher, except in the case of brief quotations embodied in critical reviews and certain other noncommercial uses permitted by copyright law.

978-1-365-36814-1

I Am Latasha Brown, LLC
www.iamlatashabrown.com

Contents

Introduction 1

You Can! You Will! 5

Now What? 9

How Did I Get Here? 13

Enjoy the Process 17

Trust the Process 21

The Struggle is Not Real 25

Whose Report Will You Believe? 29

Struggling Faith 33

Honoring God 37

Your True Identity 41

Discipline 45

God Wants the Best for You 49

Your Main Focus is to Remain Focused 53

It's Hard Work, but Worth It 57

Listen to God 61

What Are You Feeding Yourself 65

You've Come Too Far 69

Ask For Help 73

Train Yourself Right to Win 77

Prepare for the Transformation 81

God Chose You 85

Strive for Balance 89

Your Journey Requires Vision 93
Be Content 97
Set a New Standard 101
What a Great Feeling! 105
The Reward is Yours, It's His Promise 109
New Normal 113
Stay the Course 117
You Made It 121

Introduction

How many have heard the saying, "Your health is your wealth?" Do you believe that statement? I believe your health is your wealth when you make the changes to improve and invest in your health. It is essential to giving a long lasting, fulfilled life. The purpose of this devotional is to encourage you on your journey to a healthy lifestyle, through daily development in the knowledge of God's word. I'm sharing what helped me get through the fears, mistakes, tears, good, bad, struggles; but more so how I remained consistent by leaning on God's word. John 3:16 shows us how much God loves us, "For God so loved the world that he gave his only begotten son, that whosoever believed in Him should not perish, but have everlasting life." (NKJV) God chose me, so I decided to choose me, too.

The intent of using God's word is to help you remain positive and hopeful during your journey to a healthier, happier you. His word will help you develop Godly thoughts so you will not only remain positive throughout your journey, but you will remain consistent, and be successful in meeting your goals.

I truly believe that thoughts are things. When we are going through any journey in life, it is important to think positive. Our thoughts will become words, and our words will become actions. We have to feed ourselves with something positive every single day. A negative mind will never yield a positive life.

When I think about the saying, "Your health is your wealth," I can't help but to think about my family, my husband, my children, my parents, my grandparents, and my friends. I know how it feels to start something and quit because it's just not going the way I had planned. I know how it feels to go through the emotional roller coaster of weight loss and weight gain. I know how it feels to be stressed, hurt, bitter, broken, and the feeling of being alone, not realizing that all these factors contributed to my weight gain. From my personal experiences, I have discovered that daily devotional reading is the key to being positive and successful on this journey.

I want to share my journey with you; how I succeeded and picked myself up when I failed and wanted to give up; how I stood on God's word, when I felt like I couldn't make it and I just wanted to go back to old habits and quit; how those old habits made me feel like I was in control and I was comfortable with that.

God's word can set the tone for your day and give you inner strength to push through. When we fellowship with Him daily, He releases wonderful knowledge to us, and equips us for what lies ahead. Through devotional reading we find out what God thinks about us. He wants to give us hope and an amazing future. He reveals and reminds us of everything that we can do and that's what helps us become successful, and hopeful, on our journey to a healthier lifestyle.

When we give God control of our lives, our minds are constantly renewed and we are reminded of what we can do. This allows us to experience more joy than we have ever experienced. So many women are searching for support on their journey to become healthy, lose weight, maintain their weight loss, and find joy and happiness in their lives. This 30-day devotional will not only give you strength to get started, but to choose you, put your health first, and remain committed and consistent throughout the journey. This book is filled with scriptures, encouragement, and tips to help you keep a healthy body, mind, and spirit.

I pray that this book will draw you into a deeper fellowship with God. I pray that this book will help you lean on God, and not to your own understanding. I pray that this book will be a resource to provide you with an opportunity to develop personally on a daily basis. I pray that this book helps you achieve success and victory in your weight loss journey. I pray that this book helps you break the cycle of quitting on you, and helps push you through any obstacles that stand in your way.

Gracious Father,

Thank you for this opportunity to share my journey with your people. Thank you for your grace and mercy towards us. Lord, my prayer is for the woman who is reading this book to be encouraged to start her weight loss journey or healthy lifestyle, put her health first, and not only to get started, but to succeed in meeting her goals. Father, may she keep you as her main focus as you guide her on her journey. Give her the strength to keep going day by day. Remind her that she is more than a conquer. I pray that she leans on your word daily to get through any trials and temptations that come her way. Surround her with positive people. And may you be glorified daily. We are going to magnify you God because you are worthy.

In the name of Jesus, Amen.

Day 1
You Can! You Will!

Philippians 4:13 (KJV) "I can do all things through Christ who strengthens me."

You did it. You made the choice to start today. The day you decided to choose you. This is the day you decided to be committed to the process. Reflect on the reason you decided today is the day. When you hold onto that reason, it will help you keep pushing. Meditate on Philippians 4:13. Throughout this journey you will need strength to keep going day by day. In order for us to be strong, we have to lean on God's word.

He doesn't expect us to be strong. In fact, He knew we would be weak. We think we can do many things on our won. However the moment we get weak, we want t quit. When we lean on God's strength, we are reminded that we can do all things - not some things - but all things through Christ who strengthens us. When we stand on God's word, quitting will never be an option. On the days to come, remember that He is our strength and, through Christ, we will succeed.

I remember the day I chose me. That day, I made a decision to put my health first. That day, I decided I was worth it, and that my health matters. That day, I realized my family needed me. I remember when I was going through the last trimester of my pregnancy with my last baby. I was experiencing preeclampsia. My blood pressure was so high.

The doctor kept telling me that I will most likely be on medication for hypertension. That moment scared me.

After I gave birth to my baby and released to work out, I worked hard to lose weight. However, what I had failed to realize is that it's would take more than exercise. I had to control what I ate. Nutrition is the most important aspect to a healthy lifestyle. The right nutrition leads to weight loss. My body grew weak. I dreaded my follow up appointment with the doctor, which only revealed that my blood pressure was still going up. Even though I lost a few pounds, it did not change the results of my blood work.

All I could think about is how my mom and dad were faced with being on medication for hypertension since their early 20's. I remember the day I decided to put my health first. I had received a phone call from my mom. She told me that she was tired of being sick. The doctors could not control her blood pressure. No matter what medication they prescribed her, it was still high. In addition to having high blood pressure, she was a diabetic. I cried. After hearing that news, I knew it was time for me to get serious about my health. I prayed with my mom. After we prayed, I asked God to use me to be an example for others. I prayed and asked God for strength to be committed to this process.

I knew getting healthy it would be challenging. I also knew I would not be able to do this alone. I didn't want to accept the doctor was telling me that my health issues were genetic. Since my mother and father had been diagnosed with hypertension, I would most likely be diagnosed as well. I could have accepted his report. I could've gone along with that diagnosis and could be taking medication today. But I refused. I decided to fight for my life. I decided to choose me!

Today, I want to remind you that you are created in God's image. You don't have to accept and claim everything people say about you. There is another way. It's God's way. I am thankful that you chose today as your day to get started. You are worth it. Remind yourself daily that your health matters and you will put your health first. Remember that you can do all things through Christ who strengthen you. Seek God throughout your journey. You will be lifted and encouraged to fight for your life. Take it one day at a time and, remember, this is for you. Set your goal and prepare to demolish it.

Gracious Father,

Thank you for today. Thank you for giving your child the courage to get started. Continue to give her strength throughout her journey to keep going. Remind her that she is not alone, that you are with her. May peace and joy be upon her throughout her journey.

In Jesus Name, Amen.

Day 2
Now What?

Hebrews 11:1 (KJV) "Now faith is the substance of things hope for, the evidence of things not seen."

You have set your goal and started your journey. Whether you are doing this to lose weight, get healthy, or get in shape, you have started and that's enough to praise God for. The first thing you have to do when starting your journey is to have faith. Let's talk about faith and why it's important for success. See, on this journey, you will be hopeful that you meet your goals, lose weight, and stay on course. You will be anxious to see the results. Even when you feel like you're not making progress, you must have faith that you will get there.

Do you know what a mustard seed is? It's one of the smallest seeds on earth. When you ask God for help on this journey, all you need is faith the size of a mustard seed that he will help you get through any temptations, setbacks, and/or mistakes, and he will turn it all around for you. Having faith will give you assurance. Whether or not you notice the results, keep leaning on God and following his guidance. In due season, you will reap the rewards of being committed to yourself.

Faith is continuing through the process even when the numbers on the scale do show up. Faith is eating a salad instead of fries because you know that it's going to improve your health. Faith is parking at the far end of the parking lot because you know this would help your heart. Faith is when you keep pushing because people want to see you quit and you don't want to continue.

I remember thinking, okay, now I have made up my mind to start and be committed, now what? And it seems like everything came my way to distract me. I wanted to make an excuse about how eating healthy was going to be so expensive. I couldn't afford to buy groceries for me and my family. I was so used to eating out. It was quick and cheap. Then it hit me. I realized if I want to see change, I would have to make changes. I had to have faith and believe that God would make away for me if I trusted him.

You can't have faith and doubt. If you have included God in your journey, doubt shouldn't exist. I must admit, many times I would doubt myself. You see, when you're on this journey, you have to remind yourself why you started. Whether or not your spouse is not making the changes with you, or your kids still want pizza, cake, and nuggets, there's no excuse to doubt yourself or the process. You have to do this for you, first. You have to be the change you want to see in others, be an example, and have faith that, eventually, they will jump on board.

You're probably asking yourself, "Now what?" Keep it simple. Don't over complicate the process. I researched the internet for healthy foods and recipes. I began to write my grocery list, separate from my family's list. I started making small changes, such as drinking more water, eliminating sweets, eating healthier snacks, preparing my meals, and setting time aside to pray and meditate. You must have faith that God is giving you strength through this journey, strength to avoid distractions, temptations, and to remove the excuses. The excuses come. But the questions you have to ask yourself are, "Will you trust the process? Will you lean on God before you give in?"

Lean on God's word. Talk to him when you feel your commitment and consistency to the process wavering. When you lean on God, your faith will increase. Knowing God's word will give you hope that he wants you to take care of the body that he gave you. Even though, previously, you may not have been successful with your weight loss or healthy lifestyle, you have to have faith that this time will be different. You have a partner. You are not doing this alone. God has your back.

Today, I want to remind you that you're going to be great because God is on your side. God is your strength. He is your motivation. God is your help. God wants us not only to be spiritually fit, but physically fit, too. His word says in 1 Corinthians 10:31 (NIV), "So whatever you eat or drink or whatever you do, do it all for the glory of God." He gave us this body, so we must take care of it. So He will be glorified.

Gracious Father,

Thank you for today. God continue to give me strength on this journey. Help me to avoid temptations and help me to eat the right foods that are nourishing to my body. Bring wisdom and truth to my mind regarding the journey. Bring restoration, balance and well being as you allow this transformation to flow out of me, giving me courage and hope. And bless my efforts with sustainable results. God, I look to you as my supporter, comforter, and helper.

In Jesus Name, Amen.

Day 3
How Did I Get Here?

Jeremiah 29:11 (NIV) "For I know the plans I have for you, "declares the Lord," plans to prosper you and not to harm you, plan to give you hope and a future."

Isn't it wonderful to know that we have God on our side? He wants us to prosper in our lives. He doesn't want us to be around anything or anyone that may cause harm. He wants to give us hope. In order for God to give us hope and a future, we have to address our past, let go, and let God. In order for us to move on, break free, and experience a breakthrough during our journey, we have to find out how we got to where we are.

What's so great about God is that, no matter how we got here, he never left our sides. His word reminds us he will never leave us. Have you ever just wondered how in the world I got here? How did I gain so much weight, and how in the world am I going to lose it? I've been there. I have felt this way several times.

I remember after I had my baby, I weighed 208 pounds. I lost 20 pounds, and life happened again. I got busy to the point where I put my health on the back burner and gained 17 pounds. One day I got on the scale and it showed 205 pounds. I sat in the bathroom crying like a baby, thinking here I go again.

I was so uncomfortable being overweight. My self esteem was low. I wasn't in a good mental place. I put things on hold because I didn't feel comfortable and I knew I needed to be better, not only mentally but physically, for my family. I knew that I had traveled this journey alone and was unsuccessful but, with God on my side, I was confident I could do this.

How do we get here? Is it just life, taking care of the family and putting ourselves on the back burner? Is it our career, working several hours, and not taking the time to take care of ourselves? Is it a bad break up or divorce? Is it our health declining due to a medical condition? Are there issues from the past that lead to mistrust and emotional instability? Is it death of a loved one?

All of these issues, if not visited diligently, given to God, and gain closure, add stress on our lives. This is how we get here. With God's love working in our hearts, we can overcome these issues we hold. We can heal, emotionally, and it allows us to travel this journey easier. Surrender it all to God. Allow him to heal those wounds, while we continue to remain focused and break free.

Many factors contribute to being overweight, like lifestyle, not getting enough sleep, not exercising, not eating properly, and some medical conditions. Social factors, such as poverty, can have a huge impact on your health. Psychological and emotional issues can also lead people to overeat and not exercise as much.

Many times, we get to this point due to lack of self worth or self esteem. In order to remain successful on this journey, we must get to know ourselves. Not only get to know ourselves, but know what God thinks of us. We get so caught up in what the world thinks and we forget to seek God's direction for our lives. We get so caught up taking care of everyone else, that we fail to take care of ourselves. That's how we get here. We are so concerned about pleasing others, that we don't focus on pleasing God.

I want to remind you that God has a plan for you. God is your hope. God wants you to prosper in every area of your life, including your health. He will keep you encouraged on this journey. Jeremiah 29:11 reminds you that, with God, you have hope for your life and your future. Own who you are in Christ and enjoy the journey. Allow God to get close to you, and use your journey to inspire someone else.

Gracious Father,

I thank you for not giving up on me. Even when I fail to take care of myself, when I don't believe in myself, and when my circumstances get in the way, I can rest knowing you are always there, and you care for me. Help me change the way I view my circumstances. Help me to obtain closure so that I can be successful in my transformation process. Help me to make the necessary lifestyle changes needed for my body, mind, and spirit.

In Jesus Name, Amen.

Day 4
Enjoy the Process

Phillipians 4:6 (NKJV) "Be anxious for nothing, but in everything by prayer and supplication, with thanksgiving, let your requests be made known to God."

Never be so anxious to lose weight that you forget to enjoy the process. Take the time to learn about yourself and your body. Take the time to learn how to adjust to this new lifestyle. Don't rush it. Take your time to create healthy habits. Don't get so caught up on the numbers on the scale.

I remember I would be so anxious to see the scale go down. And when it did not, I was so disappointed. What I did not realize is the entire weight loss journey and healthy lifestyle process takes time. Not my time, but God's time. When you include God on this journey, you have to trust God's timing. God doesn't want us to be anxious for anything. He wants us to lean on him for everything.

I can remember getting caught up with wanting to see the numbers on the scale go down when I started this journey. I didn't realize I needed to take time to enjoy the process. When you choose to live healthier and lose weight, there are many factors that will play major roles in making changes. Learn to focus on the whole journey, not the number on the scale. When I would focus on the number, I would get so upset that I felt like it wasn't working. I constantly wanted to give up and quit. You have to look at the big picture. The scale may not show the number you want, but you are now eating cleaner. That's a huge step!

The scale may not show the number you want, but your clothes are fitting looser and you feel better.

Get to know yourself during this process. Find out what healthy foods you enjoy, such as fruits, vegetables, healthy snacks, and lean proteins. Learn how to make all the things that you like, but making them a healthy way. Start looking for healthy recipes and have fun with cooking and baking healthy, tasty treats. Keep a journal of what you like, experiment with different foods, write down recipes, take pictures, and have fun.

I love to cook. And, I love to eat. During this process, I learned to eat to live, and not to live to eat. There is a difference. Before, I would wake up ready to eat breakfast, and it wasn't a healthy one. While at work, I would be anxious to go to lunch so I could drive to get something fattening to eat. I would eat even though I knew I wasn't hungry. And, I would be so ready for seconds before my food would digest.

Now, I take the time to prepare my food, understand the ingredients I use, and take the time to actually enjoy the flavor my food, instead of rushing like it's my last meal.

Get in the habit of praying and asking God for guidance and direction. God will lead you. Be thankful for the small steps and strides you make on this journey. Once you start enjoying the process, the number on the scale will not be as important. Of course you want to see some results, and you will if you continue to stay the course and enjoy the process.

Be thankful for the changes that you have made. Remind yourself daily that God is with you on this journey. Take the time and acknowledge God throughout your day. Pray for wisdom and knowledge, because there is so much to learn about weight loss and living a healthy lifestyle. On this journey, we are forever learning about nutrition, healthy weight, foods, fitness, and factors that contribute to our health that will help us succeed.

When we make our requests known to God, he hears all of them. He gets us through each step of the journey. When we pray and ask God for guidance, he will give it to us. I remember, I would pray and ask God to help me stay on task with my healthy lifestyle daily. I would ask God to help me avoid temptations. At the end of the day, I would thank him for being by my side. I realized that if God wasn't by my side, if he didn't hear my request, I may have chosen to eat a burger instead of grilled chicken, fries instead of a salad, or maybe a piece of cake instead of an apple.

When you learn to enjoy the journey, it becomes rewarding. Praise God when you make those small changes. Praise God when you make those healthy choices. Praise God when you see the scale go down, when it goes up, or doesn't move. Praise God for another day and giving you a chance to try again. Don't be anxious but be thankful and joyful that you are making the changes to a healthier and happier you.

Gracious Father,

Thank you for another day you have given me on this journey. Thank you for guidance on this journey. Lord, continue to give me strength on this journey. Help me to learn to enjoy the process and find foods that are nourishing to my body and that are tasty. God, help me to make healthy choices and avoid any temptations that may come my way daily. Comfort me throughout the journey and allow me to rest in you.

In Jesus Name, Amen.

Day 5
Trust the Process

Galatians 6:9 (KJV) "And let us not be weary in well doing; for in due season we shall reap, if we faint not."

I can recall when I first started. I fell off a few days, feeling like this was not working for me. I would weigh myself and the scale would go up and down. I felt like a failure. I thought to myself, I have changed many things and I am not seeing any progress. I had begun to question the process. I would see others losing weight, meeting their goals, and looking great. Then, I would look at myself and see no results.

You must understand that this is for your health. Yes the goal may be to lose weight, but understand that the ultimate goal is to be healthy and trusting the process is what's most important. How do you trust the process? Include God on the journey. Acknowledge him and ask him for strength daily. That's how you trust the process. There will be days when it will be hard. Other days will be easier. But, with God, it's all possible.

Trusting the process means you are not measuring yourself to anyone else's progress. This is your journey. Many times we tend to look at others and think they are doing a great job or it's going good for them. They are seeing results but why am I not seeing results. When we take our eyes off of God and his promise to never leave us, we tend to compare our success to the success of others. We grow weary because we think that our outcome should be the same as someone else's. God promises to be with us. He knows our weaknesses, and, through him, we will have strength to keep going. We never have to measure ourselves to anyone else.

Everyone's experiences are unique to their journey. Believe me, if it were easy, everyone would be living a healthier lifestyle. Trust the process. Trust that all the changes that you are making will pay off. Trust that every day you acknowledge and surrender it all to God, that he is right there with you. God will never fail you. In due season, you will see the fruit from trusting the process.

Even though it seems hard at times, it will be rewarding. Think about how you are going to feel three months from now. Think about how, if you stay consistent to the process, your body going to transform. These are some of the rewards you will reap, if you stay committed to the process.

Remain focused. Remind yourself daily that this is for your health. You are making the necessary changes so that you can live a healthier, happier life. God wants you to be faithful to the process. You can't quit when the results you seek are not happening as fast as you want. If you quit, do you truly trust the process? No. You are giving up before you get a chance to experience the transformation. Stay committed to the process.

I want to remind you to focus on you and your journey. Don't ever be weary for wanting better for your health, doing well on the journey, putting yourself first, and being faithful to the process. When you trust the process, and trust that God is with you throughout your journey, in due season, in God's timing, you will reap the rewards from all of your hard work. You have to keep going.

Gracious Father,

Thank you for this journey. Thank you for being with me, caring for me, being my stronghold. Lord I ask that you continue to give me strength. Give me peace that surpasses all understandings. Help me to remain focused and not compare myself to anyone else. Lord, I surrender all to you, my health, my goals, my mind, and my body. Lord, renew my mind and give me hope for the future. Renew my strength so I won't grow weary in doing well.

In Jesus Name, Amen.

Day 6
The Struggle is Not Real

1Corinthians 10:13 (NKJV) "No temptation has overtaken you except such as is common to man; but God is faithful, who will not allow you to be tempted beyond what you are able, but with the temptation will also make the way of escape, that you may be able to bear it."

Many times you will hear others say, I can't be on any diet, I like to eat. People may look at what's on your plate and say I bet that's a struggle to eat that light. Or, what diet are you on now, you are barely eating. Some people may say to you, you are going to struggle with losing weight eating like that, you are starving yourself, or why are you always working out. You have to surround yourself with positive people. It's not about a diet. It's not about starving yourself or working out all the time. It's about eating healthier, portion control, and being in the best shape of your life, mentally and physically.

If you surround yourself with negative people that question your journey, you will find yourself attempting to justify your actions to people who only understand from their level of perception. Then, you may question your own actions. Never allow the opinion of others make you feel like this journey is a struggle. You already know God will help you with temptations. Some people try to distract you only because they feel intimidated by what you are doing.

People would say to me, "You are always trying some new diet, detox, or trying to eat healthy." Others would say, "Why don't you just be happy with yourself?" Or, "You are only going to lose the weight and gain it back. Aren't you tired of struggling with your weight?" And I had to remind myself that I am on this journey because I no longer wanted to settle. I no longer wanted to live an unhealthy life, and I am doing this for me.

Don't get caught up on being concerned about what you're doing. God is your encourager. God is your motivator. He is your comforter. Find peace in God when others doubt you or your journey. You don't have to explain yourself to anyone. Continue to be faithful to the process and trust God. Never forget that God is with you and for you. It doesn't matter who is against you. This journey is yours.

Your relationship with God and your daily prayers will help you fight negativity and temptations. Allow God to defend you. People will bring up your past and failures, but you have to tell yourself that your past will never determine your future. This time you have given God access and, through God, you will never fail.

People can and will tempt us. 1 Corinthians 10:13 reminds us that no temptation can over take us. Never worry about struggling on this journey. God is so faithful. He will provide what we need to be successful. Even when you feel like you are struggling, begin to rejoice God. Rejoicing during the struggles will produce endurance. Endurance will give you the power to withstand.

God will not let you be tempted beyond what you can handle. Don't get distracted by temptations, comments, or doubts from others. Only you and God know your goals. God wants you to remain focused on him, so you can endure the process. Others will not understand your journey. It's not for them to understand. God is there for you to lean on and put your cares upon. He wants you to have a healthy mind and body, and most of all God wants you to be happy, even if it means avoiding some people and some things.

Gracious Father,

Thank you for allowing me to get through temptations and negativity. Thank you for reminding me that the struggle is not real. Lord, I lift you up today. When I lift you up, I will be lifted. Help me to magnify you through all negative thinking. The more I allow you in, the smaller my challenges become on this journey. The more I magnify you Lord, the more I am able to ignore those who come against me.

In Jesus Name, Amen.

Day 7
Whose Report Will You Believe?

Mark 11:24 (NKJV) "Therefore I say to you, whatever things you ask when you pray, believe that you receive them, and you will have them."

For anything that you start, sometimes it's hard to give God control. I knew that when I asked God for help, it would be hard to remove myself and surrender all to God. I have lost count of how many times I have started the process of eating healthier and losing weight, and then quit because I didn't see what I wanted to see on the scale. I allowed life to distract me and went back to my old, unhealthy ways.

I had to start believing God's report. I prayed and asked God for help. I knew I couldn't do this alone. If I asked God for help, I had to start believing that he would do what I asked of him.

Remind yourself that you are not alone. God will help you defeat the things that you tell yourself. He will help you defeat fear. He will help you defeat discouragement. Speak to the mountains that stand in your way during this journey. Become confident in the power of God.

We have to speak to the issues that are hinder our weight and health problems, even the medical conditions that stand in our way. We have to start rebuking the reports the doctors tell us. We don't have to ignore them, but continue to make the necessary changes and stand firm on God's word. Don't get discouraged when the doctor comes in with his report. Speak boldly, that you are healed and walk in that manifestation of healing.

When the doctor tells you that you are overweight or obese, believe that God is working. You already prayed for help and, in due season, you will be at the proper weight. There's no need to claim obesity over your life. Don't stay in that area of discouragement because of other's reports. Know that God has plans for you. He has plans for you to prosper in your health.

Believe God's word. Let go of the negative strongholds in your life. Stop saying you can't because the doctor has prescribed you medication. God's word says you can. Stop limiting yourself by saying you can only do some things due to your health and weight issues. God says you can do all things. Stop saying you are alone or you don't have anyone supporting you on this journey. His word says he will never leave you, so you are not alone. Stop saying you are weak and tired. Maybe you had a long day at work and you don't feel like exercising. God says he will strengthen you. Whose report will you believe?

On this day, I want you to believe in God's report. Stop living in unbelief. Nothing grows there. Your unbelief will keep you mentally tormented. You will battle with wanting to do the will of God or doing your own will. In order to prosper and be in good health, you will have to believe that you will receive everything you asked in prayer of God for your journey.

Gracious Father,

This is the day that you have made. I will rejoice and be glad in it. I praise you today Lord. Continue to help me on this journey. If I mess up, help me to learn from my mistakes and keep moving forward. Help me to pay attention to all signs that show I am moving in the right direction for my health. I praise you for all signs of progress I make. You are my rock and I depend solely on you.

In Jesus Name, Amen.

Day 8
Struggling Faith

Joshua 1:9 (NKJV) "Have I not commanded you? Be strong and of good courage; do not be afraid, nor dismayed, for the Lord your God is with you wherever you go."

Often times we struggle with having faith in ourselves on this journey. We struggle with sticking with it. We struggle with staying committed. We struggle with trusting that it will work. Many times it's because of the fear of failing. I remember telling myself numerous times that I wouldn't lose the weight, that I wouldn't be successful. How could I struggle with my faith, if God is with me? The only way I would struggle with my faith, is if I wasn't obedient to the Holy Spirit that abides in me.

I had to really dig deep to understand why I struggled with my faith during this journey. I realized that much of my struggling faith stemmed from trust and emotional issues. My perception of truth had been that I was overweight and didn't want to confront my weight issues. Instead, I wanted to just push it under a rug and be comfortable with it. It was too painful to accept it.

The real truth is knowing what is true by faith. Faith allows us to have trust and confidence in something. When you operate by faith, you will have complete confidence that when you make the necessary changes and take control of your health, being overweight will no longer be an issue.

I had to check my relationship with God. There will be times where you will struggle in your faith. That is when you need to increase your time with God through prayer, meditation, and studying His word. In order for our faith to increase, it is imperative that we have consistent fellowship with God. You may not trust a complete stranger, but the more you open up to them, get to know them, and see them in action, you start trusting and believing what they say. If God is a stranger to you, you will not believe what he says in His word or believe his promises. That is why we struggle with our faith. The only way you will have faith and know what God's promises are for you, is to spend more time with Him and get to know him.

God wants us to be healthy. He wants the best for us. The world, our flesh, and the devil will distract us. We must be consistent in our prayer life and with our talks with God. This will remind us of what Christ has done for us. Romans 10:17 states, "So then faith comes by hearing, and hearing by the word of God" (NKJV). Our faith is built up by hearing God's word, by being reminded of how much God loves and cares for us. If God loves us, we should love ourselves just as much. And, by loving ourselves, we should want to take better care of ourselves as well. If that means making changes in our daily lives, then that's what we have to do.

Don't be ashamed of having struggling faith. In order to overcome it, you have to admit it. When you hide it, your struggles become barriers that will prevent growth and transformation. It is necessary to surrender all to God. Give God complete control over your life. When you give God control, He shows you how much he loves you through your weaknesses and struggles, and he still wants to use you.

I want to remind you, that throughout your journey to be healthier, you can work through your struggles. You can face them and allow God to work in you. Yes, the process takes hard work, lots of effort, and some resistance. Having faith is not always easy and God knows this. As you include Him, lean on Him daily with your questions. And in seeking understanding, you will have faith that you can do this. God wants you to give him all your concerns and doubts. Be strong and have courage. God is with you wherever you go. You are truly in good hands.

Gracious Father,

Today I honor you. I lift you up with praises. God I ask you to forgive me. God I am crying out to you today because I know you are listening. I celebrate you today. I know that every trial and struggle that I experience on this journey will produce patience, cause me to grow closer to you, and allow me to depend on you for my daily needs. Bring me to a deeper level of knowing just how much you love me. Fill me with life and power that is from you to help me be strong on this journey.

In Jesus Name, Amen.

Day 9
Honoring God

1 Corinthians 6:19 (NKJV) "Or do you not know that your body is the temple of the Holy Spirit who is in you, whom you have from God, and you are not your own?"

1 Corinthians 6:19 helped me shift my focus from losing weight, to getting healthy and honoring God with my body. When you put too much focus on losing weight, being a specific weight, and on the scale, it can cause you to get discouraged. Your main focus should be your health, and knowing that God wants you to be healthy. God created you in his image. This allows you to shift your focus to care for yourself.

Let's be real. God doesn't care about our weight. When people look at the outside, God looks at our hearts. He doesn't care whether we are skinny, if we are the "ideal" size. He created us in His image, not man's image. God cares about the fruit that we bear, such as love, joy, peace, patience, kindness, goodness, faithfulness, gentleness, and self control. When behaviors, thoughts, and emotional issues hinder the fruit that we bear, it concerns God.

Many weight and eating issues come from negative thoughts and behaviors. We tend to use overeating and eating disorders to hide from emotional pain. For me, being overweight was a manifestation on the outside of what was happening inside. I became a mother at an early age. I was scared. I was lost. I had to raise my daughter by myself. I began to work myself to death, or at least that's how it seemed, just to make it, and I stopped caring about my appearance and my health.

The real issue is not about being a certain size or weight, but about being a good steward of your body. Stewardship means to manage and care for something. When you are a good steward of your body, you can remove anything that hinders you from bearing fruit. You have to be humble and pray.
Recall David's prayer in Psalms 139:23-24 (NKJV), "Search me, O God, and know my heart; Try me, and know my anxieties; And see if there is any wicked way in me, And lead me in the way everlasting." With God's help, you can gain both wisdom and balance on this journey.

Learn to include God on your journey. Build your health through God's Word and wisdom. Seek God for guidance with your eating habits and behaviors, along with disciplining your body with a routine of regular exercise. When you do these things, your weight will take care of itself. You must shift your focus. Don't depend on the scale. Meditate on God's grace, goodness, and his love for you. It will lead to the renewing of your heart and mind, which will inspire change. Acknowledge that God created you in his image. He knew you before you were born, forming every part of your body, and making you wonderful. You should want to honor God by taking care of your body.

God is our greatest comforter, our greatest encourager, and greatest motivator. When we show God that we are making daily changes in our behavior, this shows true repentance. God also knows that we will make mistakes. He has plans in place to help us recover from the bumps and mistakes that we will encounter. We don't have to get discouraged when we don't meet our goal, or we fall short. However, we can learn from our mistakes and propel forward. The great thing about including God is He teaches us the right way, and leads us in the right direction. Never give up on yourself.

Gracious Father,

I honor you today because you are worthy. God, I ask you to renew my heart and mind on this journey. Help me to focus on my health, and remind me that I am created in your image, no matter what people say, I am wonderfully made. God help me honor and glorify you with my body. Help me to be mindful of what I eat and drink, so that in all things it is pleasing to you. God help me with any thoughts or behaviors that are contrary to your word and hinder me from bearing fruit. Lord I thank you for this journey. I will magnify you forever.

In Jesus Name, Amen.

Day 10
Your True Identity

Philippians 1:6 (NKJV) "being confident of this very thing, that He who has begun a good work in you will complete it until the day of Jesus Christ."

On this journey, you have to hold fast to your confidence in yourself. I knew the best approach for me on this journey was through God. You see, I tried it my way for a long time and failed. I knew that all things are possible with God. Not some things, but all things. Through God, I knew that I would find joy and peace on my journey. Anything that disrupts peace and takes away joy is of concern of God. I could rest assured that he would be in the midst of it all. I knew that I needed God in order to be able to fulfill my purpose for which He created me.

We have to seek our true identity through Christ. Our aim is to walk as Jesus walked. We can never compare ourselves to Jesus, but we strive to walk like Jesus did. Through Christ, we have received the abundance of grace and the gift of righteousness that reigns through Jesus. In contrast, I remember how I struggled with emotional eating. I would feel that certain foods had control over me. I felt powerless to change some eating habits which lead to me gaining weight. When I found my true identity in Christ, I began to give God control over my life and my health, and gained victory.

During my journey, I would cry out to God when I was weak, when I was tempted. I confessed my struggles to God. I would seek God for daily help through prayer, and be open to allow Him to lead me in the direction He wanted for me. God will help eliminate all the habits that destroy our health. Through prayer and meditation, I learned to appreciate my body as being a temple of the Holy Spirit, created by God. This process is not an overnight process. It's a continuous effort to remain in fellowship with God.

I reflect back to when I was overweight. I had to examine myself and my thoughts. Being overweight was due to improper eating habits and not focused on doing my Father's will. When we include God on our journey, he will restore us in the right relationship with food. Food should never control our lives. God created food so that we can enjoy it. We are supposed to enjoy its natural flavors. It is supposed to give us proper energy, strength, and help repair and rebuild our bodies. Allowing food to control us is not pleasing to God.

On this journey to a healthier lifestyle, we have to learn through, Godly principles, to eat with self control and wisdom. We must be mindful of the food we buy, considering carefully what we eat, and how we prepare our foods. We can truly respect and appreciate our bodies by controlling the foods we put in them.

Once you are able to control the things you eat, you will see the results. You will begin to notice that you are being less tempted with the things you use to eat. You will see your body transforming. You will look fitter and healthier than you ever have. When you get to know your true identity, and be confident that the good work God created in you will help you complete this process, you will enjoy yourself and the process it took to get you there.

Gracious Father,

Thank you for creating a good work in me, and bringing out my true identity. Thank you for being my strength when I was weak, thank you for building me up when I was broken. God I trust you with my goals and I know that you want the best for me. God continue to help me on my journey to do what is pleasing to you. God I don't want to live in the past, I want to run on with a great future in you. Lord I thank you for peace and joy on my journey.

In Jesus Name, Amen.

Day 11
Discipline

1 Corinthians 9:27 (NKJV) "But I discipline my body and bring it into subjection, lest, when I have preached to others, I myself should become disqualified."

As I began to increase my physical strength on my journey, I noticed that my emotional and mental strength was increased. You must learn to adapt discipline and self control. With God, you will learn to be disciplined, which simply means to be obedient to God's guidance and his will. In order to be successful and to live a healthier life, you must gain self control. Self control allows you to better manage healthy eating habits.

Self control is one of the fruits of the Holy Spirit. One aspects on this journey that I had to learn was to listen to my body and only eat when I was hungry. Many unhealthy habits and weight problems come from a disconnection from hunger signals. In order to hear the voices of the Holy Spirit, our minds and bodies will have to be able to function properly, and this includes being alert. When we over eat, our bodies are sluggish, tired, and we are not able to hear the voice of the Holy Spirit. This is when we began to make regretful decisions.

1 Corinthians 9:27 reminds us that our bodies are our servants, not our masters. When you start exercising regularly, you will notice how much stronger you have become. Our spirits do not get tired, but our minds and

bodies will. This is why we need God when we get weak. He will give us the strength we need.

Discipline will help you to improve your physical strength and endurance to physically respond to the demands of the Holy Spirit. Discipline and self control must be exercised daily in order for you to grow. Sometimes it takes a challenge in order to grow. Challenge yourself by setting new goals daily or weekly. For example, count how many times you work out in a week, and try to match or beat that number the next week. Count the number of times you ate healthy in a day and match it the next day. This will help you remain consistent. It will bring about discipline and self control. And, you will want to want to surpass that total each day or each week.

Most importantly, if exercising discipline or self control becomes an issue, ask God for wisdom on how to handle it. Discipline is the key to good health and happiness. Without discipline we become lazy. You may start out walking a little each day. And as soon as you make an excuse not to walk, you can fall back into your old habits. Without discipline, we continue to make bad food choices which can lead to certain illnesses. With daily practice and following a regular eating routine, your discipline can be improved, your habits begin to change, and you will see a difference in your life.

Self discipline contributes to you meeting your goals. A matter of fact, I believe that discipline is the most important aspect in order for you to lead a healthy life style, whether in terms of your fitness, or eating habits. Discipline will help you break bad habits, establish good eating habits, establish a regular workout routine, make healthy choices, and avoid making emotional choices.

As you go about your journey, remind yourself that improving self discipline and self control is important. Avoid temptations and distractions in order to improve self discipline. Make sure you are eating regularly and making healthy choices daily. You will become more aware of hunger issues and you will have the ability to make wiser choices. Create a healthy routine. Having a routine helps with self control. Even when you make mistakes remember God forgives you. Learn to forgive yourself, learn from your mistakes, and move forward. Remain positive.

Gracious Father,

We thank you for today. We ask for your forgiveness in any negative thoughts that we may have towards ourselves and others. God today we ask you to give us wisdom and knowledge on being discipline and gaining self control. God, as we discover new things about ourselves and our journey, we ask that you allow us to accept it and remain positive knowing that everything may not go as planned, and to be open to making changes daily. God we thank you for your guidance and your Word. May your will be done in our lives and on our healthy lifestyle journey.

In Jesus Name, Amen.

Day 12
God Wants the Best for You

3 John 2 (NKJV) "Beloved, I pray that you may prosper in all things and be in health, just as your soul prospers."

Once I began to seek God's will for my life, and take my relationship with God to another level, I realized my weight didn't matter to him, so that shouldn't be my main focus. God wants me to prosper in my health. I had to start aligning my goals with what God's plans were for me. How will I ever know what he wants for me if I don't fellowship with him through prayer, reading His Word, fasting, and meditation? I had to take my time with God seriously and be consistent. When I started leaning on God, I had a sweet reassurance about knowing exactly what he wanted for me. God wants the best for me and you, too.

There is no doubt that God wants us to be in good health. He created us. He wants us to prosper in health. He wants our souls to prosper. Taking care of our bodies and being in good health glorifies God. Our primary focus in life is to glorify God. Whatever we do, we should do it to the glory of God. If he created our bodies, he wants us to take care of them. When we spend our hard earned money on clothes, shoes, toys, bikes, and game systems, we don't want to see our children destroy them. We want our children to take care of the gifts we give them. God feels the same way. He gave us this body and we must take care of it. We cannot take care of it by filling it up with unhealthy foods and drinks that can lead to several illnesses.

As children of God, it is our responsibility to be witnesses to his goodness. Our responsibility is to spread the good news, and to share his Word. God gives us the Holy Spirit to help us to live the life he wants us to live. When we live a healthier life, we can be better witnesses. We have to model our walk with God and our faith. Our desire should be to live healthier to represent God who abides in us. Taking care of our bodies represents our temple which is God's temple.

Being in good health allows you to be physically fit to do God's work. We are created to do good things that God plans for us to do. In order to do the works for God we have to be physically able to do it. The healthier and more physically fit we are the more energy we will have. When we have more energy we are more enthusiastic about the task we are doing. How can we be a witness for God if we are always tired, sluggish, and have no energy? Often times, the foods we eat cause our bodies to shut down, and we are not able to function, focus, or do the task that we need to do for God.

When we are not physically healthy, we experience health issues which have a serious impact on our decisions and emotions. This can cause a separation from God. When our hearts are at peace it brings life to our bodies. When we give more attention to our health, we are able to be mentally alert. Good physical fitness is achieved by eating healthy and exercising. Your healthy lifestyle will help you become a great example to your family, friends, and others around you. You have to believe that your life is important. You have to want what's best for yourself, just as God wants the best for you.

Gracious Father,

We come to you humble, thankful, and seeking you for our daily walk on this journey. Lord, help us to keep our mind on our spiritual relationship with you, and let us not forget the importance of our physical health in our relationship with you. Being in good health honors and glorifies you, God. In everything we do we want to do it pleasing to you. Help us take care of our bodies physically, and not to consume things that will harm our bodies. Lord, we thank you for your support, encouragement, and comfort on this journey. You will get all the praises, worship, and glory out of our journey.

In Jesus Name, Amen.

Day 13
Your Main Focus is to Remain Focused

Proverbs 4:25(NKJV) "Let your eyes look straight ahead, And your eyelids look right before you."

When you find yourself drifting or wandering off, you lose sight of God's plans. When you are not focused on God and his plans for you, you start to lose hope. Losing hope on this journey can lead to doubt, fear, heartache, and guiltiness. Your main focus is to remain focused on God. Don't take your eye off of God, because it gives the enemy the opportunity to distract you.

The enemy will lure you in by distracting you and tempting you. When you are focused on God he will keep you on a straight path. You have to live to please God. When God is with you on this journey, it makes you resist satan's allure. He will test you to see if you are all in with God. Don't fall for his tactics. You have to continuously remind yourself that you cannot do this without God. The more you stay focused on God you remove yourself and other distractions out of the equation. It's all about God and his will for your life.

Look back over your life, the many mistakes you may have had, and the setbacks you have experienced. When I look back, many of those setbacks were because I tried to do it by myself. When I attempted to lose weight, I would lose it, just to gain it all back, because my focus was on losing weight and not getting healthy. I was focused on a quick fix, thinking that would do it for me. I never thought to include God and seek his help with my weight loss.

We have to remain focused on God so he can help us. When God is the main focus, we are able to seek him for guidance. He will put a plan in motion for us, help us through our weaknesses, and direct us on the right path. It's like traveling to a place using your memory instead of GPS. We get lost and lose track of time. When we turn on the GPS, it's like calling on God to help us when we're lost. But we can't just call on God when we are lost. We have to be consistent and call on him every day.

Some may think God has more important things to do other than help them reach their weight loss goals or to live healthier. Please remove that from your thinking. God cares about you and He wants to be part of your everyday life. Our goals are His goals, our visions are His visions, our problems are His problems, our struggles are His, no matter how simple or small we believe them to be. When we align ourselves to His will, He will help us.

Living a healthier life and losing weight doesn't have to be a constant battle. Remain focused on God. Ask him for help daily and you will be surprised how much easier and peaceful the process will be. Make it a habit to have daily talks with God. Talk to Him about your goals, your health, and your desires. God will help you focus on the right things to eat. He will help you plan your meals. Remember let your eyes look straight ahead. Don't worry about your past, your setbacks, or your mistakes. Your main focus is to remain focused on God. He's got you!!

Gracious Father,

Victory is mine, victory today is mine. I told satan to get thee behind, Victory today is mine. Lord, I thank you for helping me to remain focused. Lord, stand with me and help me keep my eyes stayed upon you. God when I am focused on you, I am confident that my goals will be met. God when I am focused on you, I don't have to worry about weapons that form against me prospering. Lord I thank you for being with me on this journey. I will continue to give you all the praises.

In Jesus Name, Amen.

Day 14
It's Hard Work, but Worth It

Matthew 11:28 (NKJV) "Come to Me, all you who labor and are heavy laden, and I will give you rest."

Let's be honest. When you try to lose weight and live a healthier lifestyle, it gets hard. To keep it real with you, you have to be a true laborer. Sometimes eating all the right foods and eliminating, or reducing intake of, all the foods you like can be heavy laden. It can be difficult.

I would be critical of myself when I wouldn't see any progress. I would stick to it, eat right, plan my meals, and then weigh myself and not lose weight, or gain a pound or two. This was so frustrating. I remember crying out to God. Don't you know when you cry out to God, he will give your body and mind the rest they need?

When we cry out to and petition God, he hears us. He sees us. You will find that he will remind you to keep going. It is hard work, especially when everyone else around you is doing their own thing, or making comments on what you are doing, or not respecting your journey. When we cry out to God, he will give you the strength to pick yourself up and keep going even when you are heavy laden, when the scale isn't moving, and when things are not going as planned.

Isn't it ironic how we will give up on ourselves at a drop of a dime, but God never gives up on us? Don't give up when you don't see the scale move. Press on. God will give you rest. He will give you peace. He will give you strength to press on. Cry out to God. He wants to give you rest so that you can keep going.

Remember those times you took days off of eating healthy, had fun, and did what you wanted to do? Then you woke up, checked the scale, and saw your weight increase 5-10 pounds. You may have felt embarrassed. I can admit I had those moments. I would be so embarrassed and ashamed. I felt like God was disappointed in me. Depression and discouragement would set in. Don't you know that God already knew that you would fall off? He wants to remind you to come to him so that he can get you back on track.

Continue to look to God and vow to press toward your goals. You have to trust that God will give you rest on your journey. Yes we mess up. Yes the scale won't move some days and, yes, it is hard work to stay committed and consistent. Guess what? It's all worth it.

Soon you will meet your goals. Soon you will make it a habit to eat healthy. Then you will make it a routine to exercise. You will be more confident in yourself. Why? It's because you cried out to God for help. You didn't depend on yourself. You leaned on God. Even though you labor hard to get to where God wants you to be, he will give you rest when you are heavy laden. Trust him.

Gracious Father,

We thank you for listening to our cries. We thank you for giving our bodies rest and our minds peace. Lord we want to continue to press on towards our goals with you. We want to be able to hear you when you call on us. We want to be able to go where you need us to go Lord. We are aware that with you, God, we can't go wrong. We want to continue with our heads lifted to see what the end has for us.

In Jesus Name, Amen.

Day 15
Listen to God

Psalm 32:8 (NKJV) "I will instruct you and teach you in the way you should go; I will guide you with My eye."

One of the biggest parts of my journey is learning to listen to God. I have been on many different diets and programs. I have joined several gyms and also had personal trainers. Have you experienced this?

On this journey, I have made it my purpose to really listen to my inner voice, the Holy Spirit, for guidance. When you ask God for help on this journey, you have to be willing to listen. Those small voices will tell you what you don't need, you've had enough to eat, or that you're not hungry. That voice will speak to you when you're exercising and it says go another mile or stay another 20 minutes. I believe God uses those thoughts and inner voices to instruct and teach us. We have to listen.

God has our best interests at heart and, with God's guidance, we can't go wrong. The beautiful thing is He wants to be part of what we do, what we eat, and what we say. This journey to a healthier and happier you will be adventurous because God is the greatest teacher.

Knowing that God is instructing and teaching me, reminds me that He knows what's best for me. If I listen to God, I am confident that I will not only meet my weight loss goal, but I will continue to eat healthy, adapt a healthy lifestyle, and maintain my weight loss. You must trust God to instruct you and teach you how to eat and how to live healthier.

Think about it. We listen to everyone else. We go to the doctor and listen to them tell us to do this and take that. We go to the nutritionist and listen to them talk about all kinds of foods and give us instructions that we find hard to follow. We go to the gyms and watch the trainers instruct us on how to use the equipment. We even listen to our family who may try to discourage us about being on this journey, AGAIN. Why not listen to God? His Word will give us everything we need to help us on this journey.

When we listen to God we also have to be obedient. When we are not obedient, we aren't quenching the spirit, mainly because we are allowing fear to take over. We listen to God's voice through the Holy Spirit and walk in obedience to his directions. When we drown God out, most times it's because we are afraid of where God is leading us or uncertainty of what he has to offer. Do you remember how miserable you were before you sought God on your journey? When you continually disregard God and his guidance, you will begin feeling miserable again and return to your addictive eating habits.

I remind you today to listen to God. Be still and listen to the Holy Spirit. Don't let fear allow you to drown out God. At times, you may be afraid of what God is doing. And what he has to offer for you on your journey may not be comfortable. God wants you to get out of that comfortable state, so you can grow. God has so much to offer you on your journey, but you must listen.

Gracious Father,

We thank you for your guidance, your instructions, your teaching. Forgive us for the times that we weren't obedient to your directions. Forgive us for allowing fear to overtake us. As we continue on, on this journey, help us God. Help us daily. Lord we want to obtain all the knowledge and wisdom that you have for us. We seek your Word and may your will be done in our lives. We magnify you God.

In Jesus Name, Amen.

Day 16
What Are You Feeding Yourself

Proverbs 23:20-21 (NKJV) "Do not mix with winebibbers, or with gluttonous eaters of meat; For the drunkard and glutton will come to poverty, and drowsiness will clothe a man with rags.

As you embark on your journey, you will find out very quickly who best to surround yourself with. Have you ever been around a group of people who tell you it's ok to cheat while you are trying to eat healthy? I have. They tell you, "Oh you can eat that or you can drink that. It's only this one time. You deserve to treat yourself." Don't be fooled. It's a distraction. You know your goals. If you keep thinking or waiting on a cheat day, it will defeat the purpose of a healthy lifestyle. Now I'm not saying that you cannot enjoy yourself. However, do it because it's something you want to do and not what others want you to do. Maybe you are not mentally ready to have a "cheat" day. Some people don't realize that something that seems small can set you back mentally and emotionally.

The word glutton describes an excessively greedy eater. I had to ask God to surround me with like minded people who were on the same journey as I was in order to remain encouraged. When it comes to your healthy lifestyle journey, you will find that everyone is not for you. Accept it. Everyone is not on the same level or journey in their lives. Everyone is not going to understand your journey, why you are eating healthy, why you'd rather exercise than hang out, why you eat at a specific time instead of going out to dinner late, or why you are always talking about your health, or your fitness. There are times you won't hear as much from others because they won't be able to relate to where you are in your life during this season. You don't have to distance yourself. As long as you have supportive friends and family, you can remain focused.

Be careful of what you feed your body and your mind. How can you prosper in your health if gluttony leads you to poverty? God wants us to have a healthy body and mind. Some people can feed you with unhealthy foods and negative words. You may find yourself getting weary and discouraged when you include certain people on your journey. Use these moments as lessons. Continue to seek God's will for your journey and he will lead you to the right people who will help you.

When we study God's word, it shows you how important our health is and the importance of taking care of our bodies. He also gives us warnings against gluttony. God forbade the Israelites from eating food that was harmful to their health. God also warns us about the foods we eat and our intake. When we consume harmful food and allow it to control our lives, it becomes idolatrous and we become dependent on it to make us feel better. This is not pleasing to God. Continuing to eat foods that are harmful can cause medical issues. Believe me, I've been there and done that. It not only leads to health risks, but becomes a financial burden.

Anything that becomes our number one focus, and starts to take the place of God, is not pleasing in his sight. God wants us to surrender to Him. People don't believe that food can become an addiction, but it can. It is important to learn to control your appetite. God wants to help you with that. Cast your cares upon God. We don't have to live off of food alone. We can also get full spiritually from the Word of God. Knowing his word will help us with balance between the physical and the spiritual. Both have to remain healthy. We have to have wisdom from God to strive for balance.

Gracious Father,

We thank you for how far we have come on our journey. God we ask you to lead us to the right, like minded people to help us during our journey. God we ask you for forgiveness for our sinful ways, even the ways we care for our bodies, and the things we feed our body. We ask you to give us wisdom on this journey to help us with balance in our lives. God we thank you, we praise you, and we lift you up.

In Jesus Name, Amen.

Day 17
You've Come Too Far

Ephesians 4:22-24 "that you put off, concerning your former conduct, the old man which grows corrupt according to the deceitful lusts, and be renewed in the spirit of your mind, and that you put on the new man which was created according to God, in true righteousness and holiness.

Praise God for how far you have come. You have to look back and thank God for where you were and how far you have come. Take this time to be thankful that you have stayed the course. You have adopted healthy habits. You are no longer focused on a certain number on the scale or a certain size, but you are taking better care of yourself and your health, and this is pleasing to God. Praise God that you have pushed through all the things that tried to set you back and, instead, leaned on God for guidance. When you think about it, it's a pretty marvelous feeling. God never fails us.

Ephesians 4:22-24 really describes our journey. See when you look back at your old habits – over eating, lack of control, not making wise choices of the foods, not caring for yourself, not taking your health serious, and not noticing the signs of eating out of balance – this was the old you. When you look back, you will see how your deceitful lust and old ways allowed you to grow corrupt.

When I look back, I noticed how I became corrupt from my old habits. I was always tired, sluggish, and sick. At that time I really didn't care enough about myself to be committed to making a change. How could I serve God if I wasn't taking care of the body that he created? I didn't have enough drive to be consistent. I wanted the results, but I didn't want to put in the work.

God always shows up on time. He will let you know when enough is enough, especially when you are tired of being tired. As soon as I leaned on God, and sought his will for my life and my health, my mind and spirit were renewed. I was reminded that He would be my strength when I grew weak on this journey. A new lifestyle was created and a new perspective on life was created. I felt like a new woman. God created a new outlook for me to reach.

I had to take off the old selfish person and put on the new person. Your journey to a healthier lifestyle or to meet your weight loss goals requires more than just wanting to lose weight. That may be your goal, but it requires more of you. You have to put aside your old habits and create new habits. God will teach and help you to be accountable. God wants our hearts. He wants us to be healthy enough to love ourselves and to bring glory and honor to Him.

Today, I encourage you to center your attention on God's will. His will is for you to be healthy, and to take care of yourself. Don't be too obsessed about your weight or your appearance, or body image. Seek God's will for your life. Continue to learn God's way for your journey. Your weight will correct itself and you will feel so much better about your complete transformation not just physically, but also mentally.

Gracious Father,

We thank you for the renewing of our bodies and minds. Thank you for standing with us on our journey. Thank you for giving us hope. Please forgive us for focusing so much on weight and body image. Thank you for allowing us to turn old habits into new ones pleasing to you. God, we thank you, we give you Glory, Honor, and Praise.

In Jesus Name, Amen.

Day 18
Ask For Help

Proverbs 12:1(NKLV) "Whoever loves instruction loves knowledge, But he who hates correction is stupid."

When you are on a journey to a healthy lifestyle, you will find enormous amounts of information available. There are programs to help you with your nutrition, meal planning, meal prepping, nutritional facts, what to eat based on your body type and blood type, and fitness knowledge. It can be overwhelming that's why it's a process. Don't try to over think things or over load yourself with information. You may want to give up because it seems like so much to absorb.

Don't be afraid or prideful to ask for help. It's ok to ask someone about preparing your food, how to meal prep, how to count calories, and even how much water you should drink. There is also plenty of information on the internet and social media that can be very helpful. God will lead you to the right resource get helpful information.

Be open, willing to accept instructions, seek guidance from knowledgeable individuals. You also have to be willing to accept correction. When you ask someone for help and they tell you that you should be doing something different, be willing to make the change. This is a learning experience. Being able to follow instructions and open to correction will allow you to go far on your journey.

Asking for help will lead you to like minded people that can help you take a different approach to your goals. Personally, I love exploring and trying new things, like new work out routines and new recipes. I also love reading about the success of others and how they learned to adapt to changes. I have applied some of them to my life. I ask tons of questions, and I even take notes. I write in my journal so I can refer back to the things I have done and changes I have made that could benefit others.

You have to remember, this is a healthy lifestyle. You are not in it just to lose weight. This is how you will live your life. With that being said, you have to be open to change because everything in life goes through change. What worked for you last year may not work for you now. You have to be willing to change or you will see your old habits sneaking back into your life.

Asking for help can also lead you to a support group. Support groups can be fun and will help you be accountable. We all know that losing weight can be difficult. For me, it is the most trying season. I have missed many activities and events because I was determined to stay committed to living a healthy lifestyle. While my friends were out eating and having fun, I would be working out or at home trying a new recipe. Forming a support group will help you be accountable, stay determined, and provide encouragement.

Gracious Father,

This is the day that you made, and we are going to rejoice for today. Lord we come to you humble and thankful. Lord we ask you to allow us to remain open during this journey. Give us the strength to not to let pride set in and stop us from seeking help. As much as you lead and guide us, we ask that you allow us to seek help in the physical realm. We thank you for keeping us accountable. And we strive to glorify you with our all.

In Jesus Name, Amen.

Day 19
Train Yourself Right to Win

1 Timothy 4:8 (NKJV) "For bodily exercise profits a little, but godliness is profitable for all things, having promise of life that now is and of that which is to come."

I had to learn the importance of training myself. The right way is to train myself to be godly. When God is not included on your journey and he is not the main focus, you may see the transformation you want, but you may turn out to be a different person. You may become a person who is not liked among others because of arrogance.

I remember watching this show about a woman who got on track with her nutrition and exercise. She lost over 100 pounds and became an inspiring success story. Along the way she also became different. Everyone said she changed for the worst. She became very conceited. She got piercings and tattoos. And although her husband supported her throughout her journey, she divorced him.

Yes, it is important to train and discipline your body physically. For lasting and real change, it's better to train by godliness. Train yourself to win by being godly. When you train by godliness, you profit in all things and it's beneficial now and through eternity.

Godliness allows you to take on the attributes of Jesus Christ. While on this journey, you should strive to not only better yourself physically but to love unconditionally, to forgive, to trust, to have joy, and selflessness. The woman on the show was only striving to look good. Her focus was only on herself. She wanted all the worldly things and rewards, and forgot about everyone that helped her along the way.

God want us to be the light of this world. Our journey should be a light for someone else, to help them, and to encourage them. God uses us which is why he wants to be a part of our journey. Many ideals of this world are about selfishness and getting ahead no matter who they have to step on or what it takes. God's way is putting His will first, and putting other people needs ahead of our own. Luke 9:23 reminds us to put our own wants and desires aside and dying to this world, by denying self, to follow Jesus.

On this journey, don't get in the habit of only focusing on yourself and your goals. Find others that need help and that would be happy to be part of your journey. Encourage others. I guarantee that you will feel more fulfilled when you shift your focus. You won't worry about your weight loss or transformation because you would be focusing on helping others. As you help others, they will become your support system and accountability partners by default. Training yourself God's way shines out into the world.

I encourage you to center your journey on God. Discipline yourself spiritually with prayer and meditation on God's word. Remain in fellowship with God. You also want to practice making decisions that are right and pleasing to

God. Put God first over all things. Most importantly, practice trusting God with your life.

Gracious Father,

Thank you for your daily guidance. God, you are a true and beautiful example of grace, mercy, and love. We praise you and give you honor daily. Please help us to train in godliness so we can shine out to the world and you get all the glory. God you are awesome and wonderful. We thank you for helping us every step of the way.

In Jesus Name, Amen.

Day 20
Prepare for the Transformation

Romans 12:2 (NKJV) "And do not be conformed to this world, but be transformed by the renewing of your mind, that you may prove what is that good and acceptable and perfect will of God."

I can admit I had it all mixed up, which is why I would never accomplish my weight loss goals. I was so jaded by what the world thought I should look like. I should be skinny, have long hair, be light skinned, but I didn't seek who God thought I should be. This world can prevent you from being successful on your journey, if you allow it. You have to include God. With God, you are destined to win.

When you are not conformed of this world, you are able to know and test God's will. The idea of being transformed is great, but being transformed God's way is beautiful. I think about how God transformed me on my journey. He took me from being overweight, eating unhealthy, not caring about my health or myself, to being healthier, happier, and more active. Even as sinners, He can take us from the lowest places of our lives and through his grace and love, transform us into something beautiful. Being transformed by God has allowed me to do what's acceptable and perfect for His will in my life.

It is easy to get caught up in the patterns of this world. This world will fill your mind with ugly lies. You can get off track by the affairs of the world, used up, and abused mentally and physically. God wants us to transform our minds from our unhealthy thoughts. You have to change the way you think about your foods, your health, your body, and your life. God will transform your old way to new ways.

In order to live healthier, you have to change the way you think about nutrition. Sometimes you think you know it all. However, in order to grow, you have to eliminate some of the things you were once told or thought, and retrain your mind to help you learn or approach things differently. It's perfectly fine to not know it all or to learn that something you once did wasn't the correct way.

I remember when I was first told that in order to lose weight, I needed to eliminate carbohydrates, fats, and oils. Then I was told that my body needed carbohydrates and healthy fats and oils to burn fat and lose weight. I thought to myself there is no way I would lose weight by adding oils, fats, and carbs. Through the renewing of my mind, and being open to accept a new way of thinking, I learned that our bodies need a certain amount of these to lose weight.

Today, take the time to transform your mind of all the old thinking. Learn to be open with retraining your thoughts with new ways that will help you. You don't have to be conformed of the patterns of the world. Once you are not focused on worldly things, you will be able to test God's will. God's will is truly good and perfect for your journey.

Gracious Father,

We lift our hands in total praise for you. Your will is good and perfect, whereas the patterns of this world is sinful. Please help us in renewing our minds so that we can look for your will for our life and our journeys. Keep our minds focused on doing what is pleasing to you.

In Jesus Name, Amen.

Day 21
God Chose You

John 15:16 (NKJV) "You did not choose Me, but I chose you and appointed you that you should go and bear fruit, and that your fruit should remain, that whatever you ask the Father in My name He may give you."

The reason you are on this healthy lifestyle journey is because God chose you. His timing is perfect and right. I think back to when I tried losing weight on my own timing, it just didn't work. Why? Well, I focused on my own agenda and did things my way. I was selfish. I thank God that he chose me because I needed God to be with me.

God wants us to bear fruit. How can we ever bear fruit operating in our old, unhealthy ways? That's why He chose us. The great thing is that although He chose us at an appointed time, it was a time where we were willing to do this Gods way. We were willing to surrender. God doesn't make you do it his way. He gives you a choice. He is ready for you when you make up your mind to surrender all to Him and do things His way.

God doesn't care if you don't have it together. He doesn't care if you don't know anything about nutrition or if you have never exercised a day in your life. God's only desire is for you to put him first. Then He will equip you and teach you. He wants to be a part of your journey. He wants to help you.

We have to be healthy so we can bear good fruit. The fruit we bear needs to be visible by the world in order for others to see our transformation. We must shine to this dying world. The fruit of His Spirit is love, joy, peace, patience, kindness, goodness, faithfulness, gentleness, and self control. The more we surrender to God and allow the Holy Spirit to reign in our lives, the more evident the fruit will be.

If you consider your old habits, would you be able to show and give love? Would it be evident in your life? I had to ask myself those questions. How could I love anyone if I didn't show myself love and take care of me? How can I represent self control if I let food control my life by over eating and being overweight?

I can admit that the fruit of the Holy Spirit wasn't evident in my life. I didn't know how to release the bitterness I was feeling and seek God for help. God doesn't want us to be bitter. He wants us to be at peace. I was ashamed. I knew I wanted to make a change, but didn't know how to be consistent.

God wants you to come to Him just as you are. You don't have to fix yourself up or 'get right' first. Let God do the fixing. Today, I want to remind you that God will accept you for you, even if you are broken, bitter, unhealthy, or overweight. He wants you just how you are. He wants to help you so you can bear fruit, good fruit that will last. He wants you to be able to ask anything and give it to you.

That's how much He loves us and cares for us. Isn't that amazing!

Gracious Father,

We kneel down before you, worship and adore you. We love you. We are thankful that you chose us and you want us to come to you as we are. Today we come to you with all our burdens, our struggles, our unhealthy habits. God we want to bear fruit that will last and remain. We thank you for your guidance. Continue to keep us in perfect peace.

In Jesus Name, Amen.

Day 22
Strive for Balance

Proverbs 11:1(KJV) "A false balance is abomination to the Lord: but a just weight is his delight."

God views health as completeness and wholeness. When you demonstrate good physical, mental, emotional, spiritual, and social conditions in your life, you are considered to be balanced and healthy. Ask yourself if you can be spiritually healthy without being physically, socially, and mentally healthy. No. It's not possible. In order to be healthy spiritually, you have to have a healthy lifestyle and a healthy relationship with God. In order to have a healthy relationship with God, you must seek his will.

As you may or may not know, I love eating pizza, cake, ice cream, and sweets. I am aware that in order to have a balanced life, I have to eat in these foods in moderation. Eating sweets everyday can increase my blood sugar level. Eating fried foods and pizza every day can cause my blood pressure to spike. When you start to experience those symptoms, you know that you are living life out of balance.

I had to plan my meals appropriately to have balance. Your life is imbalanced when you covet and put other things before God. Our old habits lead us to put unhealthy things before God and can lead us to being out of balance. In order for us to grow in Christ, we must have balance in every area of our lives. If a particular area is out of balance, give it to God and expand in God in that area. God is concerned with all aspects of our lives including:

- Physical – making sure we have proper nutrition, proper rest, and proper activities.

- Psychological – making sure we are mentally and emotionally healthy.

- Relational – making sure we are healthy enough to take care of and show love to our family, friends, and others.

- Spiritual – we are in fellowship with God, we trust him, obey him, and honor him.

We need to focus more on what God thinks and less about what others think. Having a healthy, balanced healthy life means we will not be so concerned with how others see us, but more so how God sees us. Whatever God's position is on something that should be our position not matter what others think. We have to balance God's Word with God's will for our journey. Balance gives a better perspective on things and their outcome. With our focus being on God's will and Word, we can strive to a better balanced life. On this journey, take the time to pray and meditate on his word. Have time to prepare your healthy meals. Make time for your physical activities. Schedule time to spend with your family and friends. God will help you balance your time.

Put God first and foremost on this journey. A false balance is an abomination to the Lord. Everything we need is in God's word. Know the importance in being proactive about taking preventative measures with illnesses that impact your health. Living a healthy life is a blessing. Your health determines longevity.

I encourage you to take your health serious. Our destiny is determined by our health. God teaches us the importance of how sacred our bodies are and how we should represent self care. We don't have to idolize our health. We should know that God wants us to take our health serious so that we can honor Him. Your willingness to improve daily and grow in Christ will claim your balanced and healthy lifestyle.

Gracious Father,

You have created us with a purpose and a plan. You desire for us to have a life full of joy and purpose. Please help us today so that we can fulfill the destiny you have planned for our lives. In order for us to live a balanced life, we must be obedient to your word. Lord we strive to have our priorities in place and our hearts focused on you. May your will be done in our lives.

In Jesus Name, Amen.

Day 23
Your Journey Requires Vision

Proverbs 29:18 (KJV) "Where there is no vision, the people perish: but he that keepeth the law, happy is he."

Without vision and goals on your journey, you will not be able to focus. God's word says that where there is no vision, the people perish. This is accurate because I wasn't successful on my other attempts to lose weight due to my lack of vision. I had one goal in mind and that was to be a certain weight. I didn't focus on being healthy. I just wanted to be a certain size.

We have to hold the vision and trust our process. God will give you vision on your journey. Without vision you will quit, give up, get easily distracted, or go back to your old ways. Having vision on your journey allows you to hold on to your reason of wanting to live healthier. What are you striving to achieve?

When God is the focus on your journey, you want lose sight of the final goal, which is to live healthier so that you can honor God. We start off at times, focusing on the scale, the fluctuations, and the ups and downs. I am a witness that if you focus on the scale, you will start stressing about whether it's working. Then you will feel like you are on an emotional rollercoaster. This could lead you back to emotional eating.

Being obedient to God's will and word will show you vision on your journey. A vision statement would be appropriate for your journey. It will help you to remain focused on why you want to live healthier and why you want to lose weight. Your vision statement should be visible so that you can see it and read it every day. Your vision statement should inspire you and give you direction during your journey. God's word gives us the inspiration and direction we need, so developing a vision statement should be easy for you.

Through God's word your vision statement should include the things you need to change within yourself and your life in order to get to where God wants you to be. As you start to seek God's will you will notice that your vision statement will take a new direction regarding your journey. You will start to include the things that you need to change in your life as God sees fit.

It is important that you don't lose sight of the vision from God for your journey, which is His will revealed to you for your journey. When we lose sight of God's will, this will cause us to fail. When you know the will of God and include it on your journey and in your life, you will be able to transform into a happy and content person. You will be able to be confident that your vision for your journey mirrors God's will and that you are doing what is pleasing to God.

Gracious Father,

Lord, continue to reveal to me the areas that need change and those that require restraint. Lord please strengthen me in those areas. Remind me to have vision and set realistic goals so that I won't perish. Help me with my vision statement so that I can avoid distractions and remain focused. God continue to lead and guide me as I seek your will for my life.

In Jesus Name, Amen.

Day 24
Be Content

Psalm 28:7 (KJV) "The Lord is my strength and my shield; my heart trusted in him, and I am helped: therefore my heart greatly rejoiceth; and with my song will I praise him."

Isn't it an amazing feeling when you are finally in a state of peace and happiness on your journey? It wasn't until I became content with where I was and how far I had come with God on my side, that I truly felt at peace and happy with myself. I was able to let my heart trust God. I was able to rejoice in how much He taught me and helped me with my weight issues. For all He has done I was able to break free and praise Him.

Being content allows you to relax and feel accomplished with your progress. Allow yourself to be thankful for the small things because they do matter. Think about how you changed your food choices. Think about how you started to drink more water and less sodas and juices. Think about how you started to eat fruits instead of sweets. Think about how you started to eat more baked and grilled food instead of fried food. Think about how you have become more active. Those changes will show. The bigger picture is God is smiling down on you because of those changes you made. You are taking care of yourself and that is pleasing to God.

When you are content on your journey, the balance between your emotions and your happiness will support the health of your body, mind, and spirit. The balance will manifest itself. This allows you to focus on the present and feel a sense of calmness, instead of on how much you want to weigh or how you want to look. Focus on how you feel now and how far you've come. Understand that the more you experience stress on your journey, the more it interferes with your progress.

Stress has been linked to weight gain. Be mindful of the stressors in your life. Learn how to center your mind on being content and happy. When you focus on the Lord being your strength and shield, how can you not focus on being happy? God will help you. He will give you strength that will allow your heart to rejoice. You will be able to rest and have peace on your journey with the help from the Lord.

When you focus on being healthy and spiritually fit for the Lord, it will bring a sense of contentment. Just knowing that by making those changes and taking care of your body is pleasing to God should make you happy. Don't worry that you are not seeing results fast enough. Focus on the changes you have made and wait for the Lord to help you. He hears your cries and he sees how much progress you've made.

Today, I want to remind you to be content with all the changes you've made. As you continue on your journey, focus on things that please the Spirit. This is where you will find your peace and happiness on your journey. The great thing about your journey this time is your attention and focus will be on God. This will allow you to keep pressing, be happy, to be content, and to continue on with your journey with your head held high. Believe that God is pleased with how far you have come.

Gracious Father,

We honor you today. We don't believe that you have brought us this far to leave us. Help us to live life in your ways; with thanksgiving and contentment. We long for your voice to instruct and guide us, giving us joy and peace. We know that living according to your word will give us peace and happiness on our journey. Lord help us to know how to step out from where we are and allow us to refuse to be content with anything other than all the things you have for us. Lord we love you, we thank you, and we praise you.

In Jesus Name, Amen.

Day 25
Set a New Standard

Psalm 63:5 "My soul will be satisfied as with fat and rich food, and my mouth will praise you with joyful lips."

It's time to set a new standard. In order for me not return to my old ways, I had to keep the encounters I had with God in my heart. I began to be satisfied with the path God had for me. I discovered my journey was not about me. God used me to be an example so I could help others. I knew I had to set Godly standards on my journey so I could be the light for others who were struggling to lose weight and live a healthy lifestyle.

My soul was satisfied because this time was different. I finally broke the hold that food and unhealthy habits had on me. I finally learned how to control myself from overeating. I finally was able to confront some of the issues that were preventing me from moving forward. When I realized that all I had to do was let go and let God take control, there were joyful praises out of my mouth. I felt a sense of freedom.

It was different this time because I stayed the course. I accomplished something that I thought I could never do. God always reminded me that I can do all things through Him. That's why you have to set new standards on your journey. You don't want to eat unhealthy, feel shackled to your problems, be afraid of facing some of the painful issues, or not be able to fully live life. God wants us to be free. We have to set a new standard for ourselves.

When you include God on your journey, you'll realize it is no longer about your healthy life style or losing weight. It is about God controlling your weight issues and serving him with your all. This includes putting God first, no matter what.

When you set and raise your standard, you are simply obeying God's word and will for your journey. God is concerned with the things that influence us. Our standards will not allow us to be influenced by the things of this world. We need to be careful of what we are doing and who we allow in our space so we won't go back to our old, unhealthy habits.

It is easy to go along to get along and do what others do. It is easy to hang out with a crowd of people who are eating and drinking whatever they want. God wants you to stand out and remember all the guidance and instructions he has given you. When you follow the crowd, it can cause a setback which will lead to discouragement.

Setting a new standard will give you a lifestyle of being obedient to God's word. This will lead to many blessings. When we commit to higher standards, it eliminates some of the stress we have in our lives. It eliminates the enemy's plan for us to fail. When the devil sees that we are easily distracted, he will use those distractions to get our attention and play with our minds.

Today, I encourage you to set a new standard on your journey. Set a standard that aligns with God's word and will for your life. If you want to continue to see the blessings on your journey, continue to be consistent with seeking God and his word. Continue to put God first on your journey and serve Him with your all.

Gracious Father,

Thank you for giving me hope on my journey. Thank you for giving me a new outlook to set a new standard for my life. Lord I give thanks to you. You have given me a reason to live healthier and happier. Lord I want to set standards so that I won't go back to my old ways and habits. I want to press forward to please you. Lord I thank you. I will continue to put you first on my journey.

In Jesus Name, Amen.

Day 26
What a Great Feeling!

Romans 8:28(KJV) "And we know that all things work together for good to them that love God, to them who are the called according to his purpose."

It is the most wonderful feeling to know that all things will work together for your good when you love and focus on God. Knowing that with God, it will all work out, gave me hope and purpose during my journey. This is what made my journey so rewarding. I knew that as long as I could keep God first, acknowledge Him, and seek his will, he would work it out. He would help me with my nutrition goals. He would help me with my fitness goals. And, with his help, I would live healthier and happier.

God has a purpose for us. I started to feel good about my journey because I had purpose and my purpose was bigger than me. It's a great feeling to know that all things that are great. All things that are perfect and good come from God. We don't have to worry about how we will meet our goals. If we focus on being healthy, since that is what God wants us to do, we will get there. Stay focused on God's faithfulness. He will never leave us.

When I would find myself getting anxious about not losing weight or how I felt about myself on this journey, I had to remind myself that I would get discouraged when I focused more on myself and goals. However, the moment I started giving God praise and glorifying his name, giving Him thanks and expressing how much I love Him, I was reminded that it's all going to work out for my good and for God's purpose.

Increase your faith, knowing that God will ensure all things work out for you on this journey because you love Him. Start now. Change your thoughts about yourself and what you can do and your world will change. God wants us to be positive. Trust and have faith that He can do the impossible. And with Him, we can do ALL things. Often times we limit God. We put him in the box because we don't believe in ourselves and our abilities. Keep believing that it will all work out for your good. Your health, your goals, or whatever you have given to God, it will work out for you.

When I have a bad day, may not meet my goals and fall off for a day. I remind myself to keep going and focus on God and His promises. I know it will work out for me. Don't quit or give up because of one bad day. God knows your present, your past, and your future. He has purpose for your journey and he promises you that it will work out for you. You are called for His purpose.

The things you may have planned for your journey may not work out the way you think they will. Some days you may struggle with staying on track. And guess what…you have to plan for the struggles. You can do that by living by God's word. Living by his word allows us to stand firm when things happen and knock us off track. His word will give us hope that as long as we love him. Things will work out for us. There will be days we stumble or make bad decisions but we don't have to stress or stop. We must keep going and stand on God's word.

I want to remind you to stand on God's promises. It's such a great feeling that you have purpose for your journey. If you keep running the race that God has set before you, you will meet your goals and God will be pleased with you. Continue to believe in yourself. God believes in you. God is preparing you for great things.

Gracious Father,

We bow down before you. You are present in all things. We love you. We adore you. Lord we are praying for your help. Help keep us on task and to make sure that nothing hinders us from doing the good and great work that you called us to do. Give us purpose in my journey. Allow us to focus on the good and positive things in our lives.

In Jesus Name, Amen

108

Day 27
The Reward is Yours, It's His Promise

Hebrews 10:35-36 (NKJV) "Therefore do not cast away your confidence, which has great reward. For you have need of endurance, so that after you have done the will of God, you may receive the promise.

It's all right to be confident. I had to tell myself that I can be confident because I know that God has done great things for me. I couldn't have this great change without God. When God is in the midst of it, great things will happen. God was my solution for my weight loss journey. I hope you have established that he can and will do great things for your journey. I have received the rewards for having faith in God. It is his promise that he will supply all my needs to be successful on my journey.

There were times where it got really hard for me and I would get discouraged. However, I remained confident and I endured, focusing on God's will for my life. God wants us to be confident. We will have a great reward and receive the promise if we focus on his will. All I had to do was focus on God on those days when I felt like I didn't want to continue or I would get distracted, and even tempted. I focused on God.

God is our ultimate source on this journey. We tend to run to everything and everyone else. And, we typically are confident on the different programs available to us, believing surely they will get us where we need to be. God is our source. We need to shift our confidence from everything else and be confident in God. And, with this confidence in him, we are guaranteed to get where we need to be. God will restore us and he will heal us in all areas of our lives.

God rewards us by allowing us to engage in the activities for success. Other things we seek will give us false hope and not prepare us for the overall journey. With God we can be confident and positive in knowing that we will be rewarded. We will be successful. We will meet our goals. If we follow God, we will have hope that he will make a way for us to conquer every obstacle that arises. We don't have to give up when things look hard for us. God will give us the strength to keep going, even when we don't want to.

I have not allowed circumstances or challenges, such as the scale not moving or having an off day, to discourage me. I refuse to let those things take root. I started to lean on God for wisdom and knowledge. I was becoming more confident knowing that God is faithful and asked him for help. I put it in God's hands. I stop doubting God's timing. God is still at work on my journey, all I have to do is keep things balanced. I'm never giving up on my goals because I know that I would be richly rewarded. Accept your rewards from God and be confident. The promises are yours.

I want to remind you to remain confident in God on your journey. Don't doubt the changes that God is allowing to occur in your health and your life. God knows exactly what's right for you. He will not lead you down the wrong path. And if you get off track, He will put your right where you need to be. God never promised us that this journey would be easy, but it will be worth it and be very rewarding.

Gracious Father,

We are confident in you Lord. We will not get discourage on the things we don't see or see on this journey. We trust you. Our goal is to do all things that are pleasing to you. We believe you will continue to do a great work within us. Thank you for your faithfulness on our journey. Thank you for bringing us all the way even at times we want to turn back. Keep our eyes focused on you so we can be rewarded and receive all of your promises for our journey.

In Jesus Name, Amen

Day 28
New Normal

2 Corinthians 5:17 (KJV) "Therefore if any man be in Christ, he is a new creature: old things are passed away; behold, all things are become new.

When I surrendered all to God, I knew there was going to be a change in my life. This journey has allowed me to get closer to God. Every area of my life has been positively affected. When I thought I could never lose the weight, or maintain a healthy life style in the past, there is not one thing I believe I cannot do! Why? I know God is with me every step of the way. When you are in Christ, old things are no longer tempting or attractive. Old thinking, old life style, old ways, old habits, are in the past and cannot determine what your future looks like. This is now your new normal. Get used to it.

You stuck with God and he has transformed your lifestyle, not only with your weight, but with your mindset. When God transforms you, you don't have to worry about what you can do. You know with God you can do all things. When God transforms you into a new creature, you don't have to worry about the number on the scale. He has helped you with maintaining a healthy lifestyle and living healthier will correct your weight issues. All things are becoming new, including the way you see yourself, the places you go, the conversations you have, the foods you eat, the restaurants you choose, and sometimes the people in your circle.

This is your new season. It's time to embrace the change that God has placed on your life. You don't have to worry about all the challenges you have previously faced. This time is different. I can recall when God placed his finger on me in the past. Hr chose me and, at that time in my life, I was too afraid to walk with Him on this journey. I felt like I was so messed up. The issues of my past had me in bondage. I didn't think I was worthy to call on God to help me with my weight issues. That is why I kept trying to do it on my own and failed every single time. I knew that I couldn't successfully do this on my own. I was ready for God to recreate me into the person he desired me to be.

Let me tell you, when you are in Christ, your newness, your change, your transformation is unlike any other transformation on this earth. Take a look at the caterpillar. We are similar to the caterpillar, not knowing what we will become. However, when God get's finished, just like the caterpillar, we will transform into a beautiful butterfly, God's beautiful masterpiece. You see, we didn't know that God was going to walk with us on this journey and transform our health, our bodies, our minds, and our thinking. We thought we were just going to lose weight. God gave us a whole new outlook on everything.

God gave us a whole new formula on this path that will guarantee our success. We may want to lose weight so we can look good. God will help us change our way of thinking so that we can be healthy, take care of our bodies, and do the will of God. We will have a whole new focus to stand on God's word, seek his will for all things, and do what pleases Him.

Today, I want to encourage you to embrace your new normal. You don't have to worry about the things that you've done in the past being a factor for your future. Keep trusting God on your journey. God has brought you a mighty long way, so don't allow old thoughts to distract you from God's plan. God has created you in his image. He has recreated you for his purpose. Your new normal may have shocked you because you never thought you would get here. But, praise God for all things new and praise him for the old things that are passed away.

Gracious Father,

Thank you for the new lifestyle change. This has been a wonderful change that you have graciously opened for me. I pray that you continue to lead and guide me on my journey, as I seek to become accustomed to the changes in my healthy lifestyle. I pray you remain close to me. Help me to keep my eyes fixed on Jesus. I pray that I carry all the tasks that you have given me for my journey. Lord I offer my life and journey as a living sacrifice that I be used for your glory.

In Jesus Name, Amen.

Day 29
Stay the Course

Psalm 119:2 (NKJV) "Blessed are those who keep His testimonies, Who seek Him with the whole heart."

Even after I met my goals, I knew I needed God even more. I had to stay the course with God. I had to share my story with the world, because so many people are struggling with weight issues, and what we fail to realize that our weight issues come from other issues that we don't want to face. With God he will get us through all of our issues.

You are truly blessed when you stay the course and trust God, walking boldly on the road that God revealed for you on our journey. There is so much that God has for us and he blesses us tremendously when we follow His directions. You will find yourself doing your best to seek Him daily. When you stay the course, you no longer go off on your own will. You will seek His will. You will find yourself praying daily for guidance in your food choices so that you won't fall off track. You will pray for best decisions when you fail to plan ahead.

God has prescribed to us the best life to live in his Word. He expects for us to live by his way, not our own. When we stay the course, God will guide us. Look back over your journey. In the last few weeks, you have included God in your daily routine and surrendered, keeping all of His testimonies, reminding yourself of the changes that He helped you make, reminding yourself how you called on his name when you were weak and he showed up on time, continuing to seek him with all your heart on the days to come. If God helped you then, he will continue to help you.

Staying the course with God allowed me to realize that my life is worth living. It has also given me joy and a sense of wellbeing, along with wanting to continue living healthier. Without God I know that I will not be able to do it. With Him I can continue to have confidence by seeking His guidance. There is so much encouragement in God's word for your journey.

God gives me hope so that I won't give up. This journey to lose weight was hard for me. And maintaining the weight loss is even harder. Seeking God with my whole heart during my journey allows me to stay the course. Not saying that you won't have some stumbling blocks, or you won't have bad days, but He encourages me to get back up and keep going.

Doing things that are pleasing to God – taking care of me, continuing to eat healthy, being active, and focusing on my mind, body, and soul – makes me happy. I know it makes God happy. Many people will get to their goal and stop doing what they did to lose the weight, and then go back to where they started. Some give up to soon before they can get to their goals. Stay the course. Stay consistent. Seek God with your whole heart. He will bless you and your journey.

Today I encourage you to stay the course. Make God part of your life and your journey. Seek God throughout your journey, not just for your weight loss goals or healthy lifestyle, but seek him in all areas of your life. When you acknowledge God, and value what he is doing for you, you will stay encouraged, engaged, and on course for your desired goals. The outcome will be amazing. Continue to pray, continue to seek his will, and continue to stand on his word.

Gracious Father,

We rejoice today. Our bodies are your temple, and we want to stay the course so we can continue to eat healthy and clean. Help us, Lord, to stay on path. Even after our goal is met Lord, we want to stay on course and continue to seek you daily. Lord we thank you for your faithfulness toward us even when we weren't so faithful. Thank you for the love you show towards us even when we didn't love ourselves. Thank you Lord for this journey.

In Jesus Name, Amen.

Day 30
You Made It

Jeremiah 17-7 (NKJV) "Blessed is the man who trusts in the Lord, And whose hope is the Lord."

It has been 30 days, and you've made it. You may have experienced times where you wanted to just give up, challenges may have come your way. You made it. God reminds us that no weapons that form against us shall prosper. Throughout these 30 days we trusted God and our hope was in the Lord. He never said it would be easy, but he said he would never leave us and that gave us hope.

Reflect on all the changes that you have made. I know that I would have not made the changes without God. I know that I would have not taken this serious without God. God gives us renewed hope. He gives us a reason to want to start, stay consistent, and continue. You should rejoice that you made it through the 30 days. When you make it this far, it challenges you to keep going and to create new goals and visions for your journey.

This is now your lifestyle. Each month that you stay the course, give your new goals to God, and accomplish them, be proud. Rejoice and praise God for the changes you've made. Look back to day one. How hard it was to start? Think about if you were to go back to how you were on day one, how hard it will be to start again? God didn't bring you through this journey just for you to go back. He wants you to move forward. As much as you are happy that you made it the first 30 days, God is happy that you trusted him with your journey.

When I made it through my first 30 days, I was so excited that I lost weight. I struggled with this for so long. God not only helped me stay consistent and determined so I could meet my weight loss goals but he increased my self esteem by guiding me with his Word for encouragement. God gave me the confidence that I can succeed and that I wasn't alone. He kept me focused and comforted me when I would get distracted and tempted. Most importantly, He renewed my appreciation of my body that he created, and how important it is to take care of it.

God empowered me on my journey. That is why and how I made it. He gave me a new purpose for my journey. Apply everything that you have learned throughout these last 30 days to renew your mind and change your health, not only for the better but for a lifetime. You have transformed physically, mentally, emotionally, and spiritually. Rejoice because you made it.

Where you used food to fill the space of any empty feelings, you will now seek God to fill up those empty places in your life. What a wonderful feeling that you made it with a new perspective. God is amazingly wonderful. You trusted him and he gave you hope. Now that you've made it through these 30 days, continue to go forward, set new goals, and remember everything that God taught you through his word. Hold onto your daily testimonies, so you can remember how you made it through.

Gracious Father,

We rejoice today because we made it through the first part of our journey. Thank you for allowing us to stay strong through your guidance and your word. Thank you for your encouragement and for comforting us when we were tempted. Thank you for transforming our bodies and our minds. Thank you for renewing our minds and allowing us to apply your word and will to change our health for the better. God we will continue to set new goals, we will continue to seek you, God, and trust and have hope in you.

In Jesus Name, Amen

My Story

I remember the first day I decided to start my journey. It was a visit at the doctor's office. I remember that day so clearly. The doctor checked my blood pressure and he said by 35 I would be on medication for hypertension. I was overweight, weighing 205 pounds. My blood pressure was high. I was so upset and I didn't know what to do.

I started walking. I tried changing my eating habits and lost a few pounds but I was so weak, tempted, and couldn't stay focused. I knew I couldn't do this on my own. I had to lean on God because I knew he would lead me and guide me. I knew that he would never leave me or forsake me., Most importantly, I knew that he created my body and he didn't want me to continue treating my health like it didn't matter. I knew that I needed to choose me. I had been unkind to myself for many years. God loved me and I had to learn to love me like God did.

In order for me to love myself, I had to get closer to God. I had to find his will for my life. I knew I couldn't keep putting my health on the back burner. I had a family that needed me. I had to be an example for my spouse, my children, and my family. I prayed and asked God for help, and God did just that.

I was running from so many past issues that I just swept under the rug, and used food to cover it up and make me happy. Let's be real. We may not be able to control things that happen in our lives, but we can control what we eat and how much of it we can have. When you don't control the food you eat, it controls you. I had to take back my life and live again. I could no longer live selfishly or for food. I had to live for God. I had to live my life God's way.

It was time for me to fight for my life. I was sick and tired of weight being a problem. I had tried so many programs but failed because I went in with the intentions just to lose weight and not to change my lifestyle. I allowed myself to let wrong thinking and negative thoughts about myself hold me back. I was defeated. I didn't have the strength to fight, but God gave me the strength to fight for my life and put my health first.

Thinking about my old habits really makes me sick to my stomach. At that point I didn't know better. I thought that a good program or diet would be my solution, but I was so wrong. My solution was God. My solution was to focus on God and he would lead me in the right direction on my weight loss journey.

I wanted to be happy for my husband and children. I wanted to be happy and love myself. Most importantly, I wanted to please God. I knew that in order to lose weight I had to eat healthy. I consulted many nutritionists. And I knew the importance of being active and exercising. I was battling a spiritual and emotional issue.

I know many of you may think that the perfect diet or program is what you need. How many of those programs you tried? Ask yourself did it work. It's not the program.

It's you. What's stopping you from being fully committed to that program? I had to ask myself that. It was a deeper issue than just the program at hand.

For me, it was an emotional issue and I needed spiritual healing. That's why I decided to do this differently and surrendered my weight issues and life to God. This was a battle that I knew I couldn't fight alone. As a matter of fact, it wasn't my battle to fight. I needed God every step of the way.

God showed me what I could do with Him. I couldn't do this alone. God helped me build my confidence throughout my journey. He gave me strength to keep going through the many times I wanted to quit. God showed me just how much he loved me and how much I meant to him. Once I was able to receive the love God had towards me, I was able to love myself. It's important to learn to love yourself before you lose the weight. If not, you will continue to feel the way you did about yourself after the weight loss.

I am praising God for my journey right now. Today I wouldn't trade all the unfamiliar routes God took me through to get where I am. I was so uncomfortable. There are many great programs out there, and I was successful on a great program, but I still needed God in order to remain dedicated to the program. It wasn't easy, but it was worth it. That is why I am down a total of 70 pounds. None of the diets or exercise programs can be compared to the journey with God.

Through God I discovered how to get an abundant life. It's about getting to know God intimately. God will use your weight loss journey to bring you closer to him. My journey was for God's purpose. He is calling you to get closer to Him through your weight loss journey. I was lead to use my journey to encourage others daily through God's word. His way is truly the best way. You are not alone. I hope you have found the courage to seek God for your journey to fight for your life and choose you, like God has chosen you. I leave you with this.

"The Lord is my shepherd; I shall not want. He maketh me to lie down in green pastures: he leadeth me beside the still waters. He restoreth my soul: he leadeth me in the paths of righteousness for his name's sake. Yea, though I walk through the valley of the shadow of death, I will fear no evil: for thou art with me; thy rod and thy staff they comfort me. Thou preparest a table before me in the presence of mine enemies: thou anointest my head with oil; my cup runneth over. Surely goodness and mercy shall follow me all the days of my life: and I will dwell in the house of the Lord forever."Psalm 23:1-6

May You and Your Journey Be Blessed!!

Made in the USA
Monee, IL
21 January 2021